THE *Buena Salud*™ GUIDE TO DIABETES AND YOUR LIFE

Newmarket Books by Jane L. Delgado, Ph.D., M.S.

The Buena Salud™ Guide for a Healthy Heart

The Buena Salud™ Guide to Diabetes and Your Life

The Latina Guide to Health: Consejos and Caring Answers

[all available in English and Spanish]

THE *Buena Salud*™ GUIDE TO DIABETES AND YOUR LIFE

JANE L. DELGADO, PH.D., M.S.

Foreword by Larry Hausner
Chief Executive Officer
American Diabetes Association

NEWMARKET PRESS

This book is published in the United States of America.

First Edition

ISBN: 978-1-55704-941-4 (English-language paperback)
1 2 3 4 5 6 7 8 9 10

ISBN: 978-1-55704-942-1 (Spanish-language paperback)
1 2 3 4 5 6 7 8 9 10

Library of Congress Cataloging-in-Publication Data

Delgado, Jane L.
Buena salud™ guide to diabetes and your life / Jane L. Delgado ; foreword by Larry Hausner.
p. cm.
Includes index.
Published simultaneously in Spanish under the title: Guia de buena salud™ sobre la diabetes y tu vida.
ISBN 978-1-55704-941-4
1. Diabetes--Popular works. 2. Hispanic Americans--Health and hygiene--Popular works. I. Title.
RC660.4.D45 2011
362.196'462008968073--dc22
2010041618

QUANTITY PURCHASES
Companies, professional groups, clubs, and other organizations may qualify for special terms when ordering quantities of this title. For information e-mail sales@newmarketpress.com or write to Special Sales Department, Newmarket Press, 18 East 48th Street, New York, NY 10017; call (212) 832-3575 ext. 19 or 1-800-669-3903; FAX (212) 832-3629.

Web site: www.newmarketpress.com

Design by Keira McGuinness

Manufactured in the United States of America.

Contents

The *Buena Salud*™ Series

The mission of the National Alliance for Hispanic Health (the Alliance) is to improve the health of Hispanic communities and work with others to secure health for all. This has been a major challenge because although 1 out of every 6 people in the United States is Hispanic, too often the research, analysis, and recommendations do not address Hispanic lives. As information emerges about Hispanic health, it is clear that to achieve the best health outcomes for all, we need a different approach to health care in our communities. Besides providing the best health information, we need to create a new way to think about health that blends the strengths of the Hispanic community with the latest medical and technological advances.

The *Buena Salud*™ series is designed to make that happen. Each book identifies the key factors that define a health concern, the changes that each of us needs to consider making for ourselves and our family, the most up-to-date information to live healthier lives, and the tools that we need to make that possible.

The challenge is to sort through the daily onslaught of health-related information and recognize that many of the changes we need to make to improve our health we cannot do alone. Our sense of family and responsibility to our family is one of the great strengths in our community, and it is key to improving the health system. Nevertheless, to do so we all need to work together. Whether it is an uncle, a brother, a sister, or a *comadre,* we have to help each other become as healthy as possible. This series is for you because there is so much that you can do to improve your own health and the health of others.

We are at a critical moment when we can make all of our lives better. The promise of science is before us, and we must use every bit of information to care for our body, mind, and spirit. Through the *Buena Salud*™ series, we want to be your partner in making it happen.

Foreword

Basta! With that one word, health care advocate Dr. Jane Delgado, president and CEO of the National Alliance for Hispanic Health, has issued a call to all of us to stop diabetes. In her richly realized *Buena Salud™ Guide to Diabetes and Your Life*, Dr. Delgado makes clear that "we should be saying… *basta con la diabetes* [enough with diabetes]." Like a best friend sitting and chatting at the kitchen table, she provides caring advice and wisdom.

Of course, with Dr. Delgado as a best friend, you also gain insights from one of our country's top health experts. In a clear language and voice, this book reviews the latest in the science of diabetes. It reminds us that type 2 diabetes does not always run in families and that lifestyle changes may not only prevent or help us manage diabetes, but also result in a healthier life for ourselves and our families.

This book is very personal for Dr. Delgado, as she shares with us stories of her own mother, her best friends, and her extended family. The sense of *familia* is everywhere in the *Buena Salud™ Guide to Diabetes and Your Life*. In a real sense we are all one family working together in our efforts to achieve good health.

Want to be better prepared the next time you see your health care provider? Dr. Delgado gives you questions to ask about the testing and diagnosis, medicine, and management of diabetes. Want to take control of your diabetes? The *Buena Salud™*

Guide has tools to keep track of your numbers, health care visits, and medicines. Want to live a healthier life? Dr. Delgado has a 10-Point Program for a healthier life and a guide to healthy eating that includes pleasure as a key component. You've got to love a health plan that focuses on pleasure!

I hope you will share the *Buena Salud™ Guide to Diabetes and Your Life* with your family and friends. If you or someone you love has diabetes or wants to reduce the chance of developing diabetes, this book can help you achieve a healthier life. Dr. Delgado gives us the information and inspiration to say *¡basta con la diabetes!*

—Larry Hausner
Chief Executive Officer
American Diabetes Association

Introduction

> I know all about diabetes; I have too many relatives who have diabetes. We all seem to get it. I know that I will get it, too. It is just a matter of time. —María

The good news about diabetes is that Hispanics of all ages have learned that it is a major health problem in our community. The problem is that the information about how common diabetes is in the Hispanic community has been so pervasive and negative that it has played into the *fatalismo* (fatalism) that is part of our culture. We are left feeling as if developing diabetes is inevitable. Somehow what we know about family history and genetics has misled many Hispanic men and women to believe that they are predestined to get diabetes.

What we should be saying instead is *basta con la diabetes* (enough with diabetes), because even though diabetes may be diagnosed in several people in a family, there is no single gene that causes diabetes. The data are clear that in the majority of cases, diabetes is not predetermined by our genes; it is a condition that emerges based on the choices we make as to how we live our lives.

Diabetes is not just one disease. It is the name given to many different conditions that share a common theme. Diabetes is the way our body communicates to us that something is wrong. As a result of what's going wrong in our body, we have too much glucose (sugar) in our blood, and our body needs us to make some changes in our life for our *buena salud* (good health). When we are told that we have diabetes, that is a clear signal that our body needs help in order to function properly.

In this book what I want to share with you is how to make your life better and easier. Regardless of whether you or someone you care about has diabetes or you are trying to do whatever you can to reduce the chances that you get diabetes, this book is for you. Rather than just giving you information, the goal of this book is to give you a new starting point for your life. I want to help you create a mental attitude where you feel that you have mastery and control of your body. The goal is not looking for perfection in all you do but understanding how your actions can help you either avoid getting diabetes or avoid some of the problems that unfold when you do not control your diabetes.

Part I focuses on helping you create a new framework for thinking about what diabetes is. It also provides a new understanding of what it means that diabetes is tightly connected to other disorders, such as depression and heart disease. The 10-Point Program is a life-changing plan for avoiding or controlling diabetes. Part II provides the facts about the major conditions and terms that are commonly used when discussing diabetes. It describes what is going on when you are developing or already have diabetes and what you can do about it. Part III gives you tools to help you control your health and resources so that you are always up-to-date on what is new as far as this serious illness is concerned.

Much has changed about what we know about diabetes. And while we may remember how family members treated their diabetes in the past, the new options for medicine, medical devices, and ongoing diagnostic testing have changed the nature of the disease. We have changed, too. As health consumers, we have to be more proactive when it comes to our own health care. Through our efforts, *ganas* (strong desire), and work to make our lives better, we will be able to say *basta con la diabetes.*

Part One

THE MANY FACES OF DIABETES

CHAPTER

Who has it? 1

I looked at Jeff and saw a thin man with a big smile and a great sense of humor, even though he had just been diagnosed with diabetes. How could that be right? He exercised and always kept his weight where it should be. Lately he had found himself thirsty all the time and sometimes he just had to have dessert. Is this what diabetes looks like? It was not what I expected. He was not fat. —Lucy

When Bill told that me that he had diabetes, I looked at him in disbelief. There had been none of the classic symptoms that either one of us would have recognized. His diagnosis seemed to come out of nowhere. It shocked both of us. Now we had to recast everything in our lives—how we ate, what we ate, and when we ate. We also knew that we had to get serious about increasing our physical activity. Bill searched the Internet for information. While he wanted to know everything, all I wanted to know was why us. —Alicia

Diabetes mellitus, or diabetes, is found across all communities in the United States. While the information that we have is limited to only some Hispanic communities, it clearly shows that Hispanics have higher rates of diabetes than non-Hispanic whites. Specifically, Puerto Ricans have the highest rates of diabetes, followed by Mexican Americans, and then Cuban Americans.

There is no simple way to explain what is happening with diabetes in the Hispanic community. In the 1980s and the 1990s, what little information was known about Hispanics and diabetes was based on data from Mexican Americans and information about the Pima Indians in Arizona. It was commonly believed that, since the Pima Indians had a high rate of diabetes, the rate among Mexican Americans could be explained based on the number of people who also had American Indian ancestry. This hypothesis had to be put to rest once data on Puerto Ricans became available, as Puerto Ricans had even higher rates of diabetes and only negligible rates of indigenous ancestry.

To confound researchers even further, it seems that Mexican American females who live in the United States have higher rates of diabetes than either their non-Hispanic white counterparts or Mexican nationals. So whatever is producing an increased rate of diabetes cannot be explained simply by country of origin or our genes.

What we have learned in the past decade is that the information in our genes tells us a lot less than we expected. We learned that we had fewer genes than we believed (only 21,000) and that genes could not explain who would get diabetes.

What we can be certain about, however, is that a more complete picture about Hispanics and diabetes is just beginning to emerge. While we may not know everything, we do know that the information about diabetes and Hispanics needs to be presented within a more meaningful framework. We can begin by expanding what we know about diabetes and use that knowledge to have a positive impact on our lives and our good health.

CHAPTER

2

More than sugar

I dreaded going to see my health care provider and being told to lose weight. I have always been big and did not want to be told that I had to lose weight. When my health care provider told me I had pre-diabetes and that I was on the verge of getting diabetes, I panicked. I started to work out and I carefully watched what I ate. I did not want to take medicines and I feared injecting myself. When I went back to see my health care provider, I was relieved when she told me that I no longer had pre-diabetes. All my efforts had paid off. —Elena

We love sugar and sweets. Our taste buds and brain leap for joy when we see our favorite *dulce* (sweet). Many of us celebrate that dark chocolate is actually good for our heart and our mood. For others of us, however, our body can no longer handle sugar as well as it used to, and we have to think about sweets and carbohydrates in a different way because we are now among the millions of people who have diabetes. If you include people with pre-diabetes, the number of people in the United States with diabetes skyrockets to include 1 in 5, or 57 million people.

The answer to the question "What is diabetes?" is very complex. Diabetes is not one disease, but many.

What they have in common is that the endocrine system is not working well. Here is some basic information you need to keep in mind.

The cells in our body need to have glucose (a type of sugar) to do their work. The endocrine system produces insulin that makes it possible for cells to use the glucose in the bloodstream. Insulin is a hormone that is produced by special cells (beta cells) in the pancreas. When glucose cannot be used by cells, a person ends up with too much glucose in the bloodstream. This can occur for one of two reasons: (1) There is not enough insulin being produced, or (2) even though there is plenty of insulin, something is interfering with its ability to do its job. As a result, a person with diabetes has a level of glucose in the blood that is too high. This is the major factor in the diagnosis of diabetes. Diabetes is more than simply having too high a glucose level. Diabetes is a description of what is going on in your body. The question still remains as to what causes diabetes to develop.

While we know that the different types of diabetes have different causes, we also know that, with the exception of prediabetes and the diabetes that some women get when they are pregnant (gestational diabetes), once we have diabetes, we will have it for the rest of our lives. It does not go away.

DIABETES AND OUR LIVES—NOT A CRISIS

WHEN DIABETES IS DIAGNOSED IN US, IN FRIENDS, OR IN OUR FAMILY, it may feel like a crisis. But it is not a crisis—it is something that we can and will handle.

Keep in mind that a crisis is a short-term situation, and if you have diabetes, in most cases, you will have it for the rest of your life. Being diagnosed with diabetes means that you have a new factor to consider as you make your plans. You have to learn to incorporate new behaviors into your day-to-day life and learn what to do to live with diabetes. The best approach to addressing diabetes is one that focuses on wellness. The steps you take to control your diabetes are also good for your overall health.

One of the first things we have to do is change our distorted view of what it means to have diabetes. Too often we look at how diabetes was treated in the past and we get scared. Our fears of blindness, amputations, or kidney failure frame our perception of what it means to have diabetes. And rather than motivate us to make changes, fear makes us freeze, deny, ignore, or become anxious. And none of these responses is good. So instead of taking steps to manage diabetes, we stick our heads in the sand and hope the situation will go away. This is not an approach that will serve us well. To manage diabetes, we need to take steps that will improve our health.

To get past all this negativity, we need to know that we are the masters of our bodies and our condition. To have this level of control means we need to be aware of all the actions that we can take, all the new research on treatment of diabetes, and the support systems that are available. By doing all we can in these areas, we increase the likelihood that we will live for a long time and without diabetes-related complications that can compromise the quality of our lives.

Our actions help us to proactively reduce the impact of having diabetes. As we learn to handle the ebb and flow of our life with diabetes, we are better able to mobilize personal resources and create and activate support systems. This is critical as we see how closely linked diabetes is to other conditions that are of concern.

CHAPTER

Risk factors 3

What are risk factors?

Although the risk factors for each type of diabetes are included in Part II, we first need to understand what is meant when something is identified as a risk factor. A risk factor is like an ingredient. Just because you know the ingredients doesn't mean you can reproduce that great dish you had in a restaurant the night before. You need to know more about how the ingredients all come together.

Imagine that you are in a restaurant and you're about to sip a big mug of hot chocolate. You look into your mug and smell the aroma of the chocolate and the hot milk swirling together. You think, Yummy! Then you realize that just having the same ingredients in your kitchen does not mean you will end up with the same tasty cup. That is also true for risk factors.

You also know that chocolate and hot milk do not have to go together. They can be matched with other things as well; for example, chocolate and cake or hot milk and cereal. If we just looked at these individual items—chocolate, hot milk, cake, and cereal—we could be leaving out other factors that may be important in bringing them together to make a cake, a breakfast item, or mush. If we only had a griddle, for instance, it would be difficult to make a mug of hot chocolate.

These are the same types of reservations that we must take into account when we identify risk factors or say there is a correlation between two things when it comes to our health. We end up linking items that may go together for different reasons. It is the same with risk factors. Risk factors, correlations, or connections between factors exist for many situations and conditions. However, whether or not they cause a disease or condition is often unclear. Sometimes changing one risk factor may not change whether or not you get a condition.

Making it even more difficult to know what to do, the media is filled with health stories about risk factors. The stories are often presented in a way that could make you believe that by changing just one risk factor, you can avoid getting a disease. Most of the time it may help to reduce a risk factor, but it usually does not ensure that you will not get a disease. Our bodies are not that simple.

Our human tendency is to try to explain why things happen, so we link items together as a way to understand our experience and our world based on the knowledge we have. A good example of this is how we once thought about the earth.

For centuries, people believed that the earth was flat, and all the theories that were developed had that belief as their underpinning. It was all that people knew, so every new piece of information was used to support and explain the prevailing belief. Once new information became available, it took a lot of effort to get people to accept that there was a different way to analyze the data. A new theory had to be developed. This created a lot of controversy. At one point in history, it was controversial and dangerous to say the earth was round.

A similar situation exists in relation to obesity. While it is true that excess weight is a risk factor for diabetes, we do not know how it causes diabetes. We also do not know the mechanism by which the excess weight is related to the inability of the individual to use glucose in the bloodstream. Obesity is a factor in diabetes, but it may not be the major one that makes it all come together.

More often than we like to admit, the way we connect factors together makes us see what we see. Our beliefs about connections end up distorting our perceptions rather than informing our behavior on the best way to proceed. We end up assuming that one factor causes the other when, in fact, no such causal relationship exists. At other times, we believe that if we suppress one condition, the other one will go away. How our body functions is usually more complicated than that.

To understand more about diabetes, we need to consider some of the conditions that seem to go with it. That is, we need to know some of the ingredients that seem to come together with diabetes.

Diabetes and other conditions

CHAPTER

4

DEPRESSION AND DIABETES

The facts are clear about the relationship between depression and diabetes in all communities. Researchers have documented that there is a strong connection, or correlation, between depression and diabetes. What we know about Hispanics creates even greater concern, as Hispanics are more likely to have diabetes and depression than non-Hispanic whites.

What is much harder to understand is what the link is between depression and diabetes. At most, the research suggests that depression and diabetes are coupled in some way. The challenge remains to determine why they are found together and whether or not either condition causes the other one to occur.

There is little evidence that type 2 diabetes makes it more likely that you will become depressed. What is certain is that recent research documented that about one-third of Hispanics with diabetes do have moderate to severe symptoms of depression. In this research, depression was measured by giving people a test in which they described how they felt. The

Hispanics who had diabetes and were depressed also had more symptoms and seemed to have the greatest problem sticking to their health programs. As a result of all this, it is not surprising that they also had more of the complications associated with uncontrolled diabetes. It seemed that the longer it had been since the people had been diagnosed with diabetes, the more depressive symptoms they experienced. Hispanics who were more recently diagnosed with diabetes had fewer symptoms of depression.

The strength of the depression-diabetes link is greater for Hispanic women than for Hispanic men. It seems that the men were more successful in controlling their diabetes than the women. Having the support of family was the best predictor of fewer symptoms of depression among Hispanic women.

> I take pills, I exercise, and I try to watch myself as much as I can. Sometimes it is hard to do. —Ricardo

> Alec had been so moody and short with everyone. He was always tired. He seemed to be edgy all the time, and it was getting to me. When his health care provider told him he had diabetes, I was shocked and I also felt guilty. Could his mood have been due to the diabetes? —Lorenzo

What we know for sure is that if you have diabetes and depression, as your depression deepens you will have more complications from the diabetes, more disability, and you will be more likely to die early. The more depressed people become, the less control they have over their diabetes. This finding is consistent with our understanding about how depression compromises people by making it hard for them to manage their day-to-day life.

What we do not know is the causal relationship; that is, whether one thing causes both diabetes and depression; whether diabetes causes depression; or whether depression causes diabetes. What we do know is that the presence of both makes each more difficult to manage.

Diabetes and the Heart

> I never knew that Mom had diabetes, too. Everyone was so focused on her heart that no one realized that she had diabetes that was uncontrolled. Only later did I learn how much it would have helped for her to have had her diabetes under control.

CARDIOVASCULAR DISEASE IS THE LEADING CAUSE OF DEATH AMONG people with type 2 diabetes. A major study, called Action to Control Cardiovascular Risk in Diabetes (ACCORD), was designed to determine the benefit of different types of interventions, including intensive glycemic control (A1C target levels below 6 percent). The study included 10,000 people with diabetes who were considered at a high risk for some type of cardiovascular problem. The part of the study that was looking at the benefits of intensive glycemic control was discontinued early because the people who were getting the intensive treatment strategy were dying in greater numbers than those getting less intensive treatment.

The relationship between diabetes and the heart is very complex. Excess weight, diabetes, and heart disease are linked. A person with excess weight and diabetes is at an increased risk of heart disease. However, as data on the Hispanic community were analyzed, it became obvious that something else was going on that demanded revisions to the model to explain the relationship among these key risk factors.

Although Hispanics have higher rates of diabetes and are more likely to carry excess weight than non-Hispanic whites, the rate of heart disease among Hispanics is no higher than it is for non-Hispanic whites. Somehow our risk factors of diabetes and excess weight do not produce the higher rates of heart disease that were predicted by existing models. The reason is not just genetic, since the positive health outcomes seem to decrease the longer Hispanics live in the United States.

Understanding this dynamic is so key to our understanding of heart disease that the National Heart, Lung, and Blood Institute (NHLBI) of the National Institutes of Health is conducting a $67 million study to try to untangle the connections between these risk factors.

Another factor under consideration is the increasing recognition of the role of inflammation in both heart disease and diabetes. It is hoped that the research from this emerging area will help to decipher the mechanisms by which these and other factors figure in the onset of heart disease and diabetes.

STRESS AND DIABETES

CONDITIONS THAT AFFECT THE RELEASE OF OUR HORMONES HAVE AN impact on diabetes as well. For women, the experience of stress has an immediate impact on hormones. The exact mechanism involved in this is not clear, but it is all related to how we handle stress. For men, the relationship between stress and hormones may not be as obvious. Undoubtedly, men under stress are more likely than women to have a flight-or-fight response. The body prepares for either one of these actions by increasing our level of energy and boosting the amount of energy we have available to either fight or flee.

Although there are many types of stress, the major kinds of stress are mental stress and physical stress. Each type of stress has an impact on key hormones that come into play depending on the type of diabetes that a person has. Physical stress raises blood glucose levels for everyone. Mental stress seems to raise blood glucose levels for people with type 2 diabetes. This is not as consistent a finding for people with type 1 diabetes.

When anyone is under stress, more cortisol (a hormone produced by the adrenal glands) is released. This boosts the blood sugar level and counteracts the effects of insulin. Additionally, in women the release of cortisol has the effect of increasing belly fat. This is of great concern because belly fat is a risk factor in developing heart disease.

CHAPTER 5

Life changes to make: The 10-Point Program

What I want you to do is to take what you already know, add to that the new science I just shared with you, and reconsider the things that you can and will do to live a healthier life.

Take a look at the questions below and answer each one. A "True" answer means that the statement is true least 95 percent of the time or at least 19 out of 20 times.

1.	I eat and drink for a healthy body.	☐ True ☐ False
2.	I exercise at least 5 times a week.	☐ True ☐ False
3.	I take all my medicines.	☐ True ☐ False
4.	I have a regular source of health care.	☐ True ☐ False
5.	I stay away from smoke and other toxic substances.	☐ True ☐ False
6.	I get enough sleep.	☐ True ☐ False
7.	I have healthy relationships.	☐ True ☐ False
8.	I keep a journal of my health.	☐ True ☐ False
9.	I cherish my spiritual life.	☐ True ☐ False
10.	I know how to listen to my body.	☐ True ☐ False

Now look at your answers. It is rare for someone to give all "True" or all "False" answers. Because we are all working to be stronger and healthier than we already are, most of us will have more "False" responses. So as you decide what changes to make, begin by celebrating all the areas where you answered "True," and use the information in the sections below to reaffirm the steps you are already taking and perhaps discover some new ones. Then look at all your "False" answers as guideposts that tell you the direction in which you need to go.

If you have diabetes or want to avoid the complications of uncontrolled diabetes, items 1 through 4 are your "must-do items." As you read the sections below, you will learn the latest techniques for creating and maintaining positive outcomes in all these areas. We all know what to do, and the suggestions and tools specified below will help us set the stage to do what we know we must.

Items 5 through 10 are magnifiers. They enhance the benefits of your core actions (1–4) when you do them, and when you do not do them, they diminish the effectiveness of your efforts. Look at items where you answered "False." Read the sections below and choose at least one of the "False" answers that you will work to change to a "True." When you make the decision to follow the steps below, you are moving toward a healthier you.

10-Point Program for Health

WHETHER WE WANT TO AVOID GETTING DIABETES OR WE WANT TO learn how to take better care of ourselves once we are told we have diabetes, there are basic steps we need to take to improve our health. While these steps may seem familiar, when we look at them through the lens of diabetes, it makes us refocus what we do.

1. Eat and Drink for a Healthy Body

FOR HISPANICS, FOOD IS ASSOCIATED WITH FAMILY, CELEBRATION, AND all sorts of emotions. Sometimes we eat not because we are hungry, but because the food is there and we were taught never to waste any. While this may have been the theme we used to guide our eating through parts of our life, to be healthy we need to rethink how we talk about food and the reasons we eat. Whether we are overweight, underweight, or just the right weight, eating and drinking for a healthy body will get us to our best weight. If you need to lose weight, you know it. If you need to gain weight, you know that, too. If you are the right weight, you also know that. In other words, we all know where we are and where we should be.

To have a healthy body, however, we need to adopt a new perspective. A good place to begin is to eliminate the word *diet* from your vocabulary. Diets are what people do for a while, and, more often than not, diets end up disappointing us because we did not get the desired results. Having a healthy body is a way of life that requires being engaged in making wise choices.

If you have diabetes, you know that your body does not handle sugar well. This is a problem because the cells in your body need sugar and other nutrients to thrive. Since the system in your body that is supposed to provide a steady source of sugar is not working properly, you need to do whatever is necessary to provide that reliable and ongoing source of sugar to your body. That is why you need to be thoughtful about what you eat and when you eat. You need to monitor and keep your blood glucose level in the desirable range. Thinking about what you eat requires you to gain a deeper understanding about sugar and starches.

When you eat or drink, your body breaks down what you consume into sugar and other nutrients. The sugar in many sweets, syrups, sodas, and baked goods is obvious. Those foods that are considered starches or carbohydrates also are broken down into sugar. The difference is that some starches or carbohydrates are absorbed faster than others. Sometimes it is not clear what has carbohydrates. For example, a 12-ounce (340g) beer is filled with as many carbohydrates as a slice of bread. The alcohol in beer only complicates the situation further.

The challenge is in knowing what and how much you can and should eat and drink. Since you want to avoid a sudden rush of glucose, you should eat food that is converted to glucose more slowly. The glycemic index is very helpful: It ranks food and beverages from 0 to 100, based on how fast they are converted to glucose. Food that is converted more slowly is also known as having a low glycemic index. The glycemic index tells you how fast what you eat or drink is turned into sugar. When a food has a low glycemic index, that means the conversion process for that food is slow, and that is good. When food is converted into glucose slowly, the demand for insulin is steady. When a food has a high glycemic index, that means the carbohydrate or starch breaks down into glucose quickly, causing a rapid need for insulin. Those foods that are converted quickly give you a sugar jolt and do not help you maintain a steady level of glucose.

Does having diabetes mean that you can never have ice cream or chocolate cake? Absolutely not. You just have to plan your indulgence with respect to the needs of your body and your ability to use glucose so that you have slow and steady control.

Glycemic index of selected foods and drinks

- Low glycemic index (55 or less): tomatoes, green beans, eggplant, garlic, most fresh fruit, whole-grain pasta, brown rice, quinoa, vegetables (not potatoes), beans
- Medium glycemic index (56–69): bananas, cantaloupe, well-done white pasta
- High glycemic index (70 or higher): beer, instant rice, white rice, white bread, pasta, baked potatoes, French fries

From the ACCORD trial, the major lesson is that slow and steady is best. In order to keep your blood glucose at a steady level, you need to think of your energy needs for the day. Skipping meals or binge eating makes it very hard to keep your glucose level steady. For some people, setting up a schedule of exactly when to eat and what to eat is helpful. Most people have days that are less under their control, so what will keep them eating in a healthy way is a flexible schedule. In a flexible plan, you keep in mind that you will eat smaller meals as you will be having snacks throughout the day. Generally speaking, you need to plan for 3 moderate- to small-size meals and 3 snacking meals a day. Now, that may sound like a lot of eating, but it really is not when you start to think about how you need to space out your food and drinks throughout the day. A snack is an important part of your plan. You need to think ahead as to what that snack will be. It should not be a chocolate milk shake or a bag of chips or a piece of cake or a doughnut.

Here are some eating-plan templates for tasty, satisfying meals and snacks that will help you manage your diabetes.

These are based on a diet of about 2,000 calories a day and provide some guidance for you to adapt to what you do to meet your nutritional targets.

TEMPLATE 1: IF YOU LIKE SPECIFIC FOOD OPTIONS

8:00 A.M. **BREAKFAST**
1 egg
1 piece of whole-grain toast, pancake, or tortilla
2 pieces of Canadian bacon (low sodium)
1 tab of butter
coffee

10:00 A.M. **SNACK**
1 small apple or 1/2 cup (100ml) of berries

12:30 P.M. **LUNCH**
1 1/2 cups (150ml) of mixed salad, including your choice of greens, carrots, celery, green peppers, and radishes
1/2 tomato
2 ounces (57g) of cheese or cold cuts or meat
2 tablespoons (30ml) of salad dressing

3:00 P.M. **SNACK**
1 banana

6:00 P.M. **DINNER**
1 cup (200ml) of whole-wheat pasta, brown rice, beans, or sweet potatoes
1 cup (200ml) of green vegetable
3 ounces (85g) of lean meat, chicken, or fish

8:30 P.M. **SNACK**
15 walnuts, cashews, or other unsalted nuts

Template 2: If you like to be flexible with your time and food

Breakfast
Carbohydrate, coffee, butter or cheese

Midmorning snack
Fruit or nuts

Lunch
Lunch salad or whole-wheat pasta
with vegetables

Afternoon snack
Fruit or nuts

Dinner
Hot vegetable, brown rice, beans, protein

Evening snack
Fruit or nuts

Template 3: If you like to count calories

8:00 a.m.	**Breakfast**	450 Calories
10:00 a.m.	**Snack**	150 Calories
12:30 p.m.	**Lunch**	500 Calories
3:00 p.m.	**Snack**	100 Calories
6:00 p.m.	**Dinner**	700 Calories
8:30 p.m.	**Snack**	100 Calories

You have to learn how to eat your meals to meet the demands on your body. If you have diabetes, you should remember to keep your blood glucose level targets as follows:

BEFORE MEALS

70 to 130

1 TO 2 HOURS AFTER THE START OF A MEAL

Less than 180

I know that I do not have to go into detail about what is good for you and what you should eat only on rare occasions. There is sufficient research that shows that people know what they should and should not eat—they just do not do it. To help you apply what you know, we need to return to the 10-Point Program. This new way to eat will focus on the three principles of healthy eating: pleasure, portion, and process.

Pleasure

You have to enjoy and think about what you are eating. It means that you cannot sit and eat mindlessly. You cannot inhale your food. You cannot eat just because the bells go off at the church across the street, telling you that it is noon. You cannot eat just because you are sad or happy. You have to eat because you are hungry. If you are not hungry, then you should not eat. However, to keep your blood glucose level at a desired level, you may have to have a snack later.

When you are hungry and decide to eat, you have to enjoy what you eat. Usually, the experience of eating is preferably shared with others. This means you should eat slowly and never talk with your mouth full. It means thinking about what you are eating and what the food is doing for your body.

As the food goes into your mouth, you should satisfy your taste buds. Eating is about the pleasure of indulging in different flavors and the pleasant memories that the aromas can evoke. It is not about stuffing yourself or eating food that makes your body malfunction. We have to think about eating in a new way. A buffet is not a challenge to see how high you can pile up food on one plate, but instead an opportunity to taste the different flavors available and see which ones you truly enjoy. Eat when you are hungry and stop when you are full.

Portion

This is the hardest part of eating healthy because often what we think of as 1 serving turns out to be much more. Take a typical chocolate bar. It is 3.5 ounces, or 100 grams. When you look at the food label on the back of the package, notice how many servings are included. You may think that 1 bar is 1 serving, but the food label says it is 2½ servings. While you will probably be surprised at the number of servings that are indicated on the food label, you will be glad that you checked it out. It may mean that you have to eat your treat over the next 2½ days if you want to give yourself a healthy treat rather than an overindulgence.

The most difficult part of the 10-Point Program with respect to portion is to be honest with yourself. A standard deck of cards (length, width, and depth) is about the same size as 3 ounces (85g) of meat, and a cup (200ml) is about what you can hold in your hand. This means that our portion needs to match our rate of metabolism. An athlete or a younger person may have a larger portion because his or her body uses the food more quickly than someone who is less active. As we get older, the portion that we need gets smaller.

Process

How did the food get to your plate? The less processed the better. You have to read the food label to know what is in the food you buy. You may think you are buying grape juice, but the label says that the major ingredient is apple juice. To eat healthy also means consuming no foods with trans fats, avoiding excess sodium and other preservatives, and, in most cases, steering clear of foods with ingredients whose names you do not recognize. If you want to sweeten your food, think raw sugar or agave instead of white sugar. There are so many tasty choices to enjoy: beans, brown rice, breads and pasta that are made with whole grains, fresh fruits instead of juice or juice drinks, plantains, fresh or frozen vegetables, meat that is not processed, water instead of energy drinks, fish that is sustainable, nuts, and so much more. The principle is simple: Enjoy more of what is less processed.

Use whatever helps you to remember what is healthy—food that has a low glycemic index tends to be less processed. If thinking in terms of the glycemic index seems too complicated, keep it simple—eat what is brown, green, or colorful and avoid what is white (white rice, white bread, white sugar, salt, fat, etc.).

All this is to help you remember that the purpose of eating is to provide your body with the nutrients that you need. What you eat should be driven by your new goal to eat for a healthy body. This is a good approach for everyone, since it will make both you and your family healthier. What is good for your physical health is also good for your mood.

Remember, if you think about what you eat and how your body uses what you consume, you will be able to make better choices. As an added plus, you will be able to be more comfortable when you do physical activities and keep your glucose at optimal levels.

2. Exercise for Life

MOVEMENT IS NOT ONLY GOOD FOR MAINTAINING OUR PHYSICAL health, but it seems to have a positive impact on our mental health as well. It even dampens feelings of depression.

No matter how good it is for you or how much physical activity you do at work or did when you were younger, before you start any exercise program or change your level of physical activity, you need to discuss it with your health care provider. This is very important for people with diabetes. Although the general rule is never to exercise when your urine has moderate or large amounts of ketones (as measured with a home test kit) or your blood glucose is high, it is best to talk to your health care provider about what you should do. You will want to ask you health care provider some specific questions:

- Should you check your blood glucose level before you exercise?
- Is it okay to exercise if your blood glucose level is high? How high?
- What should you do if your blood glucose level is too low?
- Is it good to have a snack before you exercise?

Talk to your health care provider about what to do if you are or will be exercising or physically active for more than an hour to see at what intervals you should check your blood sugar level or have more snacks. Since exercising changes how your body works, you also have to adjust how you make sure that you have adequate levels of glucose.

Physical activity or exercising is something we all know we must and should do. For some of us, our daily routine is so physically exhausting that at the end of the day, we are too tired to think of doing anything physical at all. That is why it is actually very difficult to exercise because it demands that we put out energy when all we want to to do is rest. But to be healthy we have to get up and do something.

What the research shows is that, regardless of how tired we may feel, to be as healthy as possible we must increase our physical activity. This is essential for our health, and there is a variety of activities we can do to make this part of our daily routine. Some people may want to dance or run a marathon and will do so. Most of us will have to find activities that are less time-consuming but that we will do on a consistent basis for the rest of our lives.

The key word is activities, in the plural. If we do the same activity at the same time every day, our body, being the wonderful adaptive machine that it is, gets accustomed to whatever we are doing and we do not seem to get as much benefit from that activity. That is why it is important to vary what we do. The challenge is to find what will work for us.

The best kind of physical activity is the one you will do on a consistent basis. Remember: When we move, we produce hormones that make us feel good and make our body work better. These are the hormones that help us improve our blood glucose levels. We need different kinds of exercise to help our body function well.

Endurance

Aerobic exercises build your heart muscle. When you do aerobic activities, your heart beats more and you breathe harder than usual. The more you do these activities, the stronger your heart and lungs become.

Strength

Muscle strengthening is about making all your muscles (those in your legs, hips, back, chest, abdomen, shoulders, and arms) stronger by lifting weights, digging in the garden, working with resistance bands, or doing sit-ups.

Since your bones are alive, you need to strengthen them, too. Those bone-strengthening exercises are whatever makes your feet, legs, or arms support the full weight of your body. These activities make your muscles push against your bones, such as dancing, walking, jumping rope, or lifting weights.

Flexibility

Stretching is key to flexibility and the ability to move your muscles without injury.

Start slow and do what you can. It helps to keep a written record of what you do so that you can see the progress that you have made or not made. The goal is simple. You have to keep all of you moving as much as possible. Moderation is key to doing whatever you do and is the best long-term strategy to keep you motivated. While there are people who thrive on extreme sports, such activities are not part of what most of us will be able to maintain.

In addition to the type of exercise you opt for, you also need to determine the best level of intensity for your physical activity or exercise. Whether your choose low intensity (walking, yoga), moderate intensity (swimming, jogging, bicycling), or high intensity (running, jumping rope, climbing stairs) will depend on you, your level of overall health and fitness, and the guidance offered by your health care provider. For most of us, a combination of different levels of intensity will be best, but even then you must learn to pace yourself. For example, if you are walking, you should be able to talk and walk at the same time. If you are too out of breath to speak, then you are walking too fast or on too difficult a course.

The key is to try to do something. So as little as 10-minute bursts of exercise 3 times a day several days a week is better than nothing. There are so many benefits to being physically active. You just have to keep doing whatever you find that you will do and remember that it also needs to be a reasonable workout.

HIGHLIGHTS OF RECOMMENDATIONS FOR PHYSICAL ACTIVITY

IN 2008, THE U.S. DEPARTMENT OF HEALTH AND HUMAN SERVICES (DHHS) released new physical activity guidelines. Ask your health care provider which activities are safe for you. All people who are inactive should gradually increase their activity levels and not begin with vigorous activity. Even if you played some sport when you were younger, you have to ease back into it if you have not done it for a while. For adults, the guidelines advise that:

- Something is better than nothing. If you are just starting a program, you should gradually increase your level of activity. As little as 60 minutes of moderate-intensity aerobic activity per week is beneficial.
- For major health benefits, do at least 150 minutes of moderate-intensity aerobic activity or 75 minutes of vigorous-intensity aerobic activity each week. The more you do, the greater the benefits to your body.
- Do aerobic activities for at least 10 minutes at a time several times a week.
- Muscle-strengthening activities that are moderate or high intensity should be included 2 or more days a week
- Be as physically active as your abilities and condition allow, as any amount of physical activity will produce some health benefits.

3. Take your medicines

Sara could not afford all her medicines. Since she took so many, she decided that she would just stop taking one of them. She narrowed her decision to whether to take the medicines for diabetes or the medicine to control her cholesterol. It was not an easy choice, but she decided to take the medicine to control her cholesterol as she did not want to have a heart attack.

THE GOOD NEWS IS THAT THERE ARE MANY TYPES OF MEDICINES TO help you control your diabetes, and sometimes you can get help in covering the cost. Your health care provider will work with you to make sure that your medicines are working the way they should. When you are prescribed medicines to control your diabetes, you must take them. That is essential to managing and controlling your diabetes. You must also take your other medicines. If you are unsure of which medicines you should take, or if you are concerned about taking too many medicines or about the cost, you must discuss this with your health care provider.

Some people may need insulin. Insulin can be prescribed in rapid-acting, intermediate-acting, or long-acting formulations. Your health care provider will give you some combination of the different types of insulin to meet your daily needs. You can get your insulin by injection or by an insulin pump. The typical insulin pump is about the size of a deck of cards and has a catheter that goes under your skin in your stomach, lower back, leg, or arm. Although Medicare Part D helps pay for insulin, it does not pay for the type that is used with an insulin pump. At one time there was a type of insulin that you could inhale, but that is no longer available.

The medicines you are taking may not be familiar to you or to your family. Your health care provider prescribed specific medicines for you to help you control your diabetes. If you feel that your medicines are making you sick, then you need to tell your health care provider. Do not stop taking your medicines just because you do not like them or because you are feeling better or because you think they are too expensive. Talk to your health care provider before making any change in the medicines you are taking. If you are having difficulty paying for your medicines or for the supplies you need to monitor your diabetes, let your health care provider know. Medicare covers many of the costs for your medicines. You can call the National Hispanic Family Helpline (1-866-783-2645) to get information on how to get help in paying for your medicines.

Some people are concerned about taking any prescription medicines because they are not natural. They prefer to take teas or other products because they don't have as many chemicals. My response is that they are all made with chemicals. Most important of all, being natural is not necessarily healthy. Arsenic is natural, but it can accumulate in your body and kill you. Whether something is manufactured or natural is not the important issue. What is important is to take the right medicines for the right reasons. This way medicine can help you stay healthy and alive.

Others tell me they feel safer taking medicines that they can buy in another country or over the counter. The reality is that if a prescription medicine is not sold in the United States, you should not take it because it has not met the strict safety standards that are in place in this country to protect you. As for over-the-counter (OTC) medicines, you should take whatever OTC medicines your health care provider has advised you to take. Both prescription and over-the-counter medicines help our bodies do their work. If you are prescribed medicines, you need to take them. If you are having a bad reaction to them, then you need to let your health care provider know so that you can be advised on what you should do.

4. HAVE A REGULAR SOURCE OF HEALTH CARE

IN ORDER TO AVOID THE COMPLICATIONS OF UNCONTROLLED diabetes, you need to have a regular source of health care. At this moment, when health care services are changing so dramatically, you need to have a health care provider you can talk to and who will listen to you. A recent study found that, even when given a diagnosis that required follow-up, Hispanics were less likely to schedule the next visit. What increased the likelihood of pursuing treatment was finding a health care provider who understood the patient's language and the culture. Take the time to find someone you trust.

If you are diagnosed with diabetes, your health care provider may have you see other health care professionals (an endocrinologist, a dietitian, a nutritionist, a certified diabetes educator) as part of the team to help you control your diabetes. In the beginning, you may see your health care provider more frequently as you learn to manage your diabetes. Your health care provider will give you information on what to do and what to expect. Make sure you or someone you bring with you take notes when you speak to your health care provider.

On an annual basis, you should get your eyes checked (by an ophthalmologist or an optometrist), have a complete foot exam (by a podiatrist), and have your teeth and gums checked. All this should be part of your regular health care routine. If you are covered by Medicare and have diabetes, Medicare will cover part of the cost of diabetes screenings, foot exams, eye tests, and appropriate treatment.

The problem with not having regular checkups is that rather than avoiding complications, you may exacerbate them. There is much that can be done in health care today, but you need to be engaged and proactive in order to benefit from the advances.

5. STAY AWAY FROM SMOKE AND OTHER TOXIC SUBSTANCES

THIS MAY SEEM LIKE AN OBVIOUS STATEMENT, BUT SOMETIMES IT IS very hard to tell what is toxic. Nevertheless, keep in mind that every time you breathe in air, your lungs and heart work together to fill the cells that do not have oxygen with the air you just took in. The oxygen-filled cells then travel throughout your body to every tissue and organ, including your pancreas, which produces insulin. If what you breathe is toxic, then that is what will fill the cells in your body.

Tobacco is an air pollutant and it is toxic. Decades of research confirm that smoking is bad for the person smoking, the people who are near the smoker, and even the people who only inhale the lingering odor of tobacco that hangs on to the smoker's clothes and hair. When you smoke, you increase your risk of having more complications from diabetes. It is getting easier to stay away from smoke as more and more places are banning smoking.

This is also why, during days when the air quality is poor, if you go outside, you are more likely to end up in the emergency room. The Environmental Protection Agency (EPA) is starting to tighten many of the restrictions on the levels of pollutants in the air. What we know for sure is that there are too many pollutants and toxic substances and that EPA keeps track of too few of them. The section on "Endocrine disruptors" (in Part II) goes into detail about the specific impacts and consequences to your endocrine system. Airborne toxics include benzene (which is found in gasoline), dioxin, asbestos, and toluene and metals such as cadmium, mercury, chromium, and lead compounds.

Keep in mind that sometimes the most hazardous particles to breathe are the ones that you cannot see. According to the EPA, there are "inhalable coarse particles" (PM_{10}, or between 2.5 and 10 micrometers in diameter) as well as "fine particles" ($PM_{2.5}$, or less than 2.5 micrometers in diameter) in the air. The fine particles are more dangerous to our health because they settle deeper in our lungs. Fine particles are so tiny that 28 of them side by side would be as thick as a strand of hair.

While the air outside is a problem, the air inside can also be a problem. Many household and office products give off gases that are called volatile organic compounds (VOCs), some of which may have short- and long-term adverse health effects. Household products that usually release VOCs include paints, paint strippers, and other solvents; wood preservatives; aerosol sprays; cleansers and disinfectants; moth repellents and air fresheners; stored fuels and automotive products; hobby supplies; and clothing dry-cleaned with perchlorethylene. That smell of fresh paint or new carpeting is not good for your health. And some dangerous indoor substances like radon have no smell whatsoever.

6. Get Enough Sleep

YOU NEED TO GET SLEEP. THIS IS DIFFERENT FROM REST OR DOING nothing. Sleep is a function that your body needs to stay healthy. When you sleep, hormones are released that are very important to keeping you healthy. When you sleep, the hormones that control your appetite are also activated. That is why people who sleep only 5 hours a night are more likely to have excess weight than those who sleep 7 to 8 hours per night. These hormones also help to make you more alert.

When you do not sleep, your body is under stress. The stress from not sleeping changes the hormones your body produces and ends up shifting your blood glucose levels from the steady level that is your goal.

People who have a sleep disorder are at a higher risk of high blood pressure, heart attack, stroke, and other medical conditions. Your body needs this time to recuperate from the activities of the day. When you sleep, your heart rate and blood pressure are reduced about 10 percent. People who do not get enough sleep do not have this reduction and compromise their health.

How much sleep someone needs varies by age: healthy adults 7 to 9 hours, newborns 16 to 18 hours, children in preschool 10 to 12 hours a day, and school-aged children and adolescents at least 9 hours. Since everyone has different needs for sleep, it is no wonder that it is so hard to get everybody in the house up and about at the same time.

But quality of sleep is as important as quantity. Do not fool yourself by saying that a siesta or a power nap is all you need to make up sleep that you missed. Short (less than 1 hour) daytime naps can only partially make up for missed sleep. In addition, by sleeping late on the weekends, you cannot make up the sleep that you lost during the week. Not only is this a bad idea, but it also has a negative effect on your biological clock.

In order to get a good night's sleep, here are some steps you can take:

- Set a regular sleep schedule.
- Do not exercise before bedtime.
- Avoid caffeine, nicotine, alcohol, and large meals before bedtime.
- Do not take naps after 3 P.M.
- Create a sleeping environment and a relaxation ritual.

Sometimes, however, you cannot sleep because you have to take the night shift. If possible, try to avoid this shift, but if you must work during these hours, here are some steps you can take to make it easier on your body:

- Increase the total time you sleep by sleeping more and adding naps.
- Use bright lights in your workplace.
- Reduce sounds during your daytime sleep.
- Cover your eyes to block out any light.
- Cover windows to reduce the light as much possible during your daytime sleep.
- Drink caffeine only during the first part of your shift.

Getting sleep is essential to being healthy.

7. MAINTAIN AND NOURISH HEALTHY RELATIONSHIPS

IT SEEMS OBVIOUS THAT HEALTHY RELATIONSHIPS ARE GOOD FOR US, and yet establishing and maintaining solid relationships is a goal that challenges many of us. Perhaps it is because some relationships become more like a habit—something we do because we have been doing it for so long. And like a bad habit, a bad relationship is difficult to change. Emotional surges, either up or down, have an impact on the blood glucose level of men and women.

To be healthy in body, mind, and spirit, we need to have relationships that support us rather than drain us. Even at the level of each cell in our body, unhealthy relationships wreak havoc because of the stress they create and the resulting change in the hormones that our body produces. That is why, if you want to delay getting diabetes or the complications of diabetes, it is important to eliminate stress from your life and maintain stable, healthy relationships.

To reduce how diabetes impacts our life, we must reduce or eliminate stress. When you think about the stress in your life, you have to remember that coping strategies and managing stress are not something you can do for a long time. They are only meant as short-term strategies. They are not meant as a way of life. The important step is to reduce or to eliminate the level of stress in your life—not just manage it.

Learning to adapt and being flexible are essential to healthy relationships and will also be key to managing diabetes. You will need to reconsider everything you and others do as part of your relationship, from fundamental routines of life like family schedules and when you eat meals to the more complex tasks of your daily life. Healthy relationships are the ones that will support your efforts to realign what you do to delay getting diabetes or to avoid the complications of diabetes if you already have it.

Reducing stress by being flexible and learning to adapt is more than a good skill; it sustains our mind and spirit. The strength to adapt to a changing situation is born from a lifelong commitment to working to improve our relationships. The ability to make these necessary changes varies greatly among individuals. Some who have a state of mind or spirit that is fragile can make change only with substantial support, such as ongoing visits to a nutritionist and other health care professionals. Others who appear more robust will still need support, but it may be of a different kind, like written materials they can consult whenever they need some encouragement.

Healthy relationships require work and nourishment. It is not all about bliss. It is also about resolving conflicts in a positive way. All healthy relationships need to have the basic ingredients of mutual respect, affection, healthy boundaries, and sharing of responsibilities. Laughter and joy are also essential to balancing out our daily lives.

Part of a healthy relationship with your partner or spouse involves sexual intimacy. Although diabetes is known to have an impact on sexual performance in men, recent research suggests that much can be done to help with the nerve damage (neuropathy) that may contribute to the problem. Men may have erectile dysfunction (ED) because of the lack of blood flow to the penis or even as a side effect of medication. Today a man is more likely to be willing to talk with his health care provider about erectile dysfunction and how to resolve it. The good news is that health care providers have a range of options that are available and will work with you to find the solution that is most effective.

Research on the sexual problems of women with diabetes is relatively recent. Most studies have focused on sexual desire, sexual arousal, orgasm, and painful intercourse. The findings are inconsistent, so the relationship between diabetes and sexual problems in women remains unclear. What has become increasingly evident is that women have psychological underpinnings to their sexual problems. What women think has a major impact on how their bodies respond sexually. The same is true for men. We are just starting to understand these important dynamics.

Depression is one of the correlates of unhealthy relationships. When relationships are not healthy, they create a situation where depression can flourish. While men and women may respond to depression in different ways, their hormones and blood glucose levels go through dramatic shifts. These shifts should be avoided, since they upset the balance that you are trying to maintain. Healthy relationships are not about *aguantando* (putting up and not complaining). That is important to remember.

The connection between depression and diabetes highlights the importance of having healthy relationships. Being depressed is associated with feeling out of control. It is not surprising that people who are depressed have problems in gaining control over diabetes. This applies to all Hispanics, both men and women.

Healthy relationships are about eliminating stress, mutual affection, and respect for each other. Those are the factors that keep our blood glucose levels steady.

8. Keep a Health Journal

MANAGING YOUR DIABETES WILL REQUIRE YOU TO KEEP TRACK OF WHAT you consume as well as your blood glucose levels. Since mood, level of stress, and depression all have an impact on your blood glucose level, it is important to keep a written record (see "About Me: On a Daily Basis" page 111). This is important information to write down on a daily basis so that you can share it with your health care provider during your next visit. Your health care provider will use the results of your tests and your record of what you have done to see if there are any patterns in the fluctuations in your blood glucose levels. This analysis will provide important information on how to proceed.

Diabetes is a condition that you will have to manage for the rest of your life. Keeping a health journal is like managing your checking account or household budget. You have to write down what you eat and when, how you exercise and for how long, how you feel at various times of the day, and so on so that you can see where you have to make changes. Your journal will also be looked at by your health care provider and others on the team to help make decisions about your progress and care.

Although electronic medical records are a growing part of our health care system, you also need to keep track of your own health. You can do this by using any system that you want, including some that you can access through your cell phone, via e-mail, or on the Internet.

Having information at your fingertips that is up-to-date about your health and the medicines you take is essential. When you are sick or in an emergency situation is not the best time to try to recall details of your health history. Having a written health record that you or others can access quickly is essential. When you go to an emergency room, be prepared to describe your health history and to list all your medicines and their doses.

You can use the tools in Part III of this book to organize and maintain your health information. These tools are designed to make it easy for you to maintain and keep all together information that could save your life.

9. Cherish Your Spiritual Life

FOR SOME REASON, THE DIAGNOSIS OF DIABETES SEEMS TO HIT US hard. And at times like that, Hispanics can rely on their spiritual life to support them. To understand and take care of ourselves, it is helpful to have faith. At critical times in life, people turn to their religious roots for strength and solace. As Hispanics, our sense of faith sustains us, regardless of our particular religious orientation or the consistency of our practice.

Faith helps to heal and restore us. The 10-Point Program understands that the goals of health and wellness extend beyond the physical. For Hispanics, health is also about *el espíritu* (the spirit).

10. Listen to Your Body

THIS IS AN ESSENTIAL SKILL FOR EVERYBODY, BUT ESPECIALLY FOR PEOPLE with diabetes. When you have diabetes, you need to maintain a stable state of being so that your level of blood glucose matches what is provided by what you eat with an assist from medicines, if they are being used. Men have to practice listening to their inner self and hearing what their body is saying to them. Women seem to have more experience at recognizing hormonal shifts. While having a glucometer makes it easy to measure your blood glucose level, men and women need to become more aware of how the body reacts to shifts in their blood glucose levels. In many ways the glucometer can help you recognize the signs your body gives when there is a problem.

You need to keep a steady and level amount of glucose in your body. When your blood glucose level is too low (a condition known as hypoglycemia), you may find that you feel hungry, shaky, nervous, sweaty, dizzy or light-headed, sleepy, confused, anxious, weak, or have difficulty speaking. You may have one of these symptoms or you may have several. But if you have diabetes, you just cannot ignore it. You should measure your blood glucose level and, based on the results, decide what to do next (see "Hypoglycemia" on page 94). You can also become hypoglycemic when you sleep. If you are sleeping, you may find that you cry out or have nightmares; sweat so much that your sheets become damp; or feel tired, irritable, or confused after waking up. Just as important is recognizing how you feel when your blood glucose levels are too high, such as being very thirsty and urinating excessively.

Be aware of changes in your body and what might have caused them. No one knows you as well as you can and should know yourself. You need to be on very familiar terms with the language that your body uses when it signals to you that things are good or not so good.

The key things for you to remember are simple, since they are the basics for healthy living for ourselves and for our families. In summary, the 10-Point Program for health encourages and supports your efforts to:

1. Eat and drink for a healthy body
2. Exercise for life
3. Take your medicines
4. Have a regular source of health care
5. Stay away from smoke and other toxic substances
6. Get enough sleep
7. Maintain and nourish healthy relationships
8. Keep a health journal
9. Cherish your spiritual life
10. Listen to your body

Part Two

JUST THE FACTS

> I've had diabetes for 20 years and I still don't know everything I should. They keep changing the rules.
>
> —Carlos

Research makes clear that diabetes is the name given to many disorders that all have in common the inability to use sugar (glucose) properly. As a result of this problem, the level of glucose in the blood is higher than it should be, as the cells cannot use the glucose that is essential for them to function properly.

What we know about diabetes and how to manage it has changed dramatically in recent years. We need to know the facts because much is changing as new types of diabetes are identified and the causes of particular types are better understood. In order to present what is most useful, what follows are some abbreviations that are commonly used, a description of diagnostic tests for diabetes, and information about the major types of diabetes.

Over the decades, the major kinds of diabetes were known by many names that were based on either the treatment that was needed (insulin-dependent or non-insulin-dependent diabetes) or the age at which diabetes was first diagnosed (adult onset or juvenile diabetes). In 1997 an expert committee of the American Diabetes Association recommended that the names for the two major types should be type 1 and type 2. The other types of conditions under *diabetes* are pre-diabetes, type 1.5, gestational diabetes, and diabetes that is brought on by specific genetic defects. Although these are covered in this section, there are other types of diabetes that are not included here because they are much less common. These other types of diabetes may stem from diseases of the pancreas (pancreatitis and cystic fibrosis), conditions that upset the production of hormones (cortisol is produced in Cushing's syndrome and cortisol works counter to insulin), medicines or chemicals that destroy the beta cells in the pancreas that produce insulin, infections (such as congenital rubella and cytomegalovirus), and an autoimmune disease of the central nervous system (stiff person syndrome). That these types of diabetes have such different causes only adds to the complexity of trying to understand diabetes. Moreover, although these are different diseases, what they have in common is that they affect insulin production or insulin use.

Finally, in addition to the types of diabetes, Part II provides information on some of the key systems in our body that are related to diabetes. Understanding how these systems work will help you appreciate how far-reaching and crucial the decisions you make about food, activity, medicines, self-monitoring, and stress management really are.

ABBREVIATIONS

ACCORD	Action to Control Cardiovascular Risk in Diabetes, a major research study that looked at cardiovascular disease and type 2 diabetes
CDC	Centers for Disease Control and Prevention
DCCT	Diabetes Control and Complications Trial
DHHS	U.S. Department of Health and Human Services; includes the NIH and the CDC
DPP	Diabetes Prevention Program
EPA	Environmental Protection Agency
NHLBI	National Heart, Lung, and Blood Institute; is part of the National Institutes of Health
NIDDK	National Institute of Diabetes and Digestive and Kidney Diseases; is part of the National Institutes of Health
NIEHS	National Institute of Environmental Health Sciences; is part of the National Institutes of Health
NIH	National Institutes of Health

Diagnostic tests

A huge problem is that one-third of people with diabetes do not know that they have it. To determine whether or not you have diabetes, you will be given one of the blood tests described below. If your test results suggest that you have diabetes, you will have a second set of tests on a different day to confirm the diagnosis. To determine if you have type 1 diabetes, your health care provider will also (1) check for ketones (compounds that are produced when your body excessively breaks down fat) in your blood or urine and (2) analyze your blood to see whether you have the special antibodies that are found in people who have type I diabetes. The following tests are used to diagnose diabetes.

Fasting Plasma Glucose (FPG) Test

When you take a fasting plasma glucose (FPG) test (see Table 1), you will be told not to eat anything for at least 8 hours. This test is used to detect diabetes and pre-diabetes. It is a convenient, low-cost test, and is the preferred test. You usually have this test in the morning.

Table 1. Fasting Plasma Glucose (FPG) test

Plasma Glucose Result (mg/dL)	Diagnosis
99 or below	Normal
100 to 125	Pre-diabetes (impaired fasting glucose)
126 or above	Diabetes

Oral Glucose Tolerance Test (OGTT)

This is used to diagnose diabetes, pre-diabetes, and gestational diabetes (see Table 2). For this test, you fast for at least 8 hours, have a fasting glucose test, drink a glucose-containing beverage (75 grams of glucose dissolved in water), and 2 hours later have another glucose test. This test is better for diagnosing pre-diabetes, but it is more complicated to do.

Table 2. Oral Glucose Tolerance Test (OGTT)

2-Hour Plasma Glucose Result (mg/dL)	Diagnosis
139 and below	Normal
140 to 199	Pre-diabetes (impaired fasting glucose)
200 and above	Diabetes

To diagnose gestational diabetes a pregnant woman will be asked to drink a beverage with 100 grams of glucose. Her blood glucose levels are checked four times during the test. If at least 2 blood glucose levels are above normal, she is diagnosed with gestational diabetes. Table 3 shows the above-normal results for the OGTT for gestational diabetes.

TABLE 3. GESTATIONAL DIABETES: ABOVE-NORMAL RESULTS FOR THE OGTT

WHEN	PLASMA GLUCOSE RESULT (MG/DL)
Fasting	95 or higher
At 1 hour	180 or higher
At 2 hours	155 or higher
At 3 hours	140 or higher

Note: Some laboratories use other numbers for this test. These numbers are for a test using a drink with 100 grams of glucose.

RANDOM PLASMA GLUCOSE TEST

This test is also also called a casual plasma glucose test, and is done regardless of when you last ate. This is the test that is commonly given at free health screenings. It can diagnose diabetes but not pre-diabetes. If your blood glucose level is 200 mg/dL or higher and you are experiencing one of several symptoms (increased urination, increased thirst, unexplained weight loss, fatigue, blurred vision, increased hunger, or sores that do not heal), your health care provider will check your blood glucose level on another day using the FPG test or the OGTT to confirm the diagnosis of diabetes.

GLYCATED HEMOGLOBIN (A1C) TEST

This is a blood test that looks back at your blood sugar level for the past 2 to 3 months. This test is a key part of your regular visits to your health care provider and the ongoing monitoring that is essential to managing diabetes.

Since June 2009 the American Diabetes Association, the European Association for the Study of Diabetes, and the International Diabetes Federation have recommended that this test be used for diagnostic purposes, too. The National Institute of Diabetes and Digestive and Kidney Diseases (NIDDK) does not recommend the use of the A1C for diagnosing diabetes.

The results from the A1C may be given in several ways—as a percentage, as an estimated average glucose (eAG) level in mg/dL or mmol/L, or as a value of mmol hemoglobin A1C/mole hemoglobin. The eAG is the easiest for most people to understand, since it uses the same measure as the glucose meter that you use to monitor yourself.

For the majority of people, the A1C is able to give your health care provider a feeling for your average blood sugar level during the past 2 to 3 months. The A1C results are inaccurate for some people, for example, pregnant women and people with an inherited variation in their hemoglobin (hemoglobinopathies). The latter is more common in people of African, Mediterranean, or Southeast Asian descent. Most people do not know they have this inherited condition.

Your health care provider will probably want you to take an A1C test at least 2 times a year. This blood test reveals what your memory may not want to disclose as accurately. In other words, while you may feel compelled to tell your health care provider that you have controlled your diabetes very well, the test will reveal whether or not you actually did so. This test is used as part of the ongoing monitoring that your health care provider will do to track how you have been managing your diabetes. Accuracy in your record keeping and reporting is very important.

If the results of your A1C are very different than what you have recorded in your daily record, or the result is greater than 15 percent, or the result is dramatically different than your last test, your health care provider may recommend additional tests to determine if there is another reason to explain the results.

For most people, the goal is for the A1C results to be below 7 percent (see Table 4). Maintaining a level below 7 percent greatly reduces the risk of certain complications of diabetes, such as loss of vision, foot ulcers, neuropathy, and kidney damage. Make sure your health care provider tells you what is the best result for you. If your results are not what they should be, your health care provider will work with you to make your plan more effective.

TABLE 4. WHAT YOUR A1C RESULT MEANS

My A1C Result	My estimated average glucose level (eAG)
5%	97
6%	126
7%	154
8%	183
9%	212
10%	240
11%	269

Test for Ketones in Your Blood or Urine

When your body does not have enough glucose, it uses fat for energy and in the process produces ketones. Although this may sound like a good thing, it is not. Ketones in your body are bad. When you produce too many ketones, you are at risk of ketoacidosis, which can kill you if left untreated. Signs of this problem include one or more of the following symptoms:

- You feel like vomiting.
- You feel weak.
- You start to breathe fast or have a hard time breathing.
- Your breath has a sweet smell.

You can also check for ketones at home using a test kit. Ask your health care provider whether you should do this.

Endocrine disrupters

ALSO KNOWN AS
endocrine modulators, environmental hormones, and endocrine active compounds

No one has mentioned anything to me about endocrine disrupters. However, I also have a mild hypothyroidism for which I am being treated. That's how I ended up seeing an endocrinologist so many years before I was diagnosed with diabetes. —Laurie

I have heard of fish that were born with both male and female sex organs or some other characteristic that was off. Do you think that whatever is doing that to the fish could have an effect on us, too? —Liz

---

Que pasa?

Endocrine disruptors are chemicals that are believed to disrupt or interfere with the hormones in humans or animals. These chemicals have bad effects on the endocrine system, the immune system, our growth and development, reproduction, and brain functioning. These chemicals are both naturally occurring (for example, the phytoestrogens that are found in some plants) or manufactured, such as pharmaceutical products, dioxin and dioxin like compounds, polychlorinated biphenyls (PCBs), DDT and other pesticides, and chemicals used to make plastic, such as bisphenol A (BPA).

These chemicals disrupt the functioning of the endocrine system. Birth control pills are an example of an intentional endocrine disruptor. They were developed to prevent pregnancy by disrupting, or changing, the monthly hormonal cycle of women.

In other cases, the disruption that resulted was not intentional, and our hormones do not work the way they are supposed to. This inability of the endocrine system to function properly may have several causes. For example, a chemical may:

1. Act like a hormone, prompting the body to respond as if it were the hormone, such as by imitating a growth hormone and getting the body to increase muscle mass.
2. Trigger signals at the wrong time, such as increasing production of insulin when it is not necessary.
3. Block a hormone from reaching the tissue where it is supposed to be, such as preventing growth hormones from reaching the cells and tissues for normal development.
4. Stimulate or inhibit the endocrine system and cause overproduction or underproduction of hormones (e.g., an over- or underactive thyroid).

Causes and Prevention

What we learn sometimes takes a lot of time, and in the interim there is much suffering. For example, from the 1940s to the 1970s, clinicians would give women who were pregnant and who had a high risk of having a miscarriage a medicine called DES (diethylstilbestrol). DES was an estrogen that had been created in the lab and was believed to be a medicine that not only would prevent miscarriages but would also help babies grow. DES was given to 5 million pregnant women. It was not until the daughters and sons born to these women reached puberty that concerns began to arise. It seemed that DES was more powerful than ever imagined. It had a negative impact in the development of the reproductive systems of the children of the women who had taken DES during their pregnancy. As the data trickled in, what emerged was a pattern of increased cases of a rare vaginal cancer among the daughters and numerous noncancerous changes in both the sons and daughters.

Given the tremendous amount of time between exposure and effect, and the amount of monitoring that is essential, scientists have a hard time making the connection between exposure to endocrine disruptors and a negative consequence. This is why the impact of these chemicals as environmental contaminants that wreak havoc on the endocrine system is considered controversial. While we have good data on the impact on animals, studies with people have been lacking. The National Institute of Environmental Health Sciences (NIEHS) has developed ways to use animal models to make predictions about human impact.

To improve what we know and to better track the impact of endocrine disruptors throughout the population, Congress established the Endocrine Disruptor Screening Program (EDSP) within the Environmental Protection Agency (EPA). This is a highly significant step, even though the program only focuses on estrogen, androgen, and thyroid hormones.

NIEHS has supported studies to determine the human health effects of these chemicals. The focus of these studies has been limited to the impact on the ability to have children (fertility) and the increases in the number of people who have endometriosis or specific cancers.

The cause of the endocrine disruptions in our environment are very specific chemicals that are increasingly pervasive in our communities. For example, PBDEs (polybrominated diphenyl ethers) are everywhere. PBDEs are a type of flame retardants used in many consumer products, such as foam cushions in furniture, carpet padding, clothing, and electronics. Today they are also appearing in salmon, butter, cheese, and ground beef. Given that these compounds are found in so much of what is around us, it is very hard to avoid exposure. In one NIEHS study, 97 percent of the women participants had measurable levels of PBDEs in their blood.

Q ***Do I have a problem?***

We all have a problem. We live in an increasingly toxic stew, but our bodies can handle some of it. We are only beginning to assess the impact of these chemicals. Perhaps the disruption of our endocrine system will also be seen as a factor accounting for some of the global increase in diabetes.

Q ***What do I do now?***

The best action to take is to know the chemicals that you are exposed to and to try to reduce the chemicals that you and your family come in contact with. This includes household cleaning products, bug sprays, paint, garden and plant chemicals, and so on.

Endocrine system

Que pasa?

Diabetes is considered an endocrine disorder, which is why an endocrinologist is often added as part of your health care team.

The endocrine system is made up of glands and hormones that are located throughout your body. Hormones are special chemicals that deliver messages to other cells so that they know what they must do. The communication that goes on between hormones and cells is unique. Each hormone has its own language that can be understood only by the specific cells the hormone enables or with which it is supposed to work. That is how hormones act with other cells to meet the needs of your body.

Specialized glands not only make the hormones we need but they also release them into the bloodstream and into other neighboring cells. These endocrine glands include the hypothalamus, the pineal, the pituitary, the parathyroids, the thyroid, the islets of Langerhans in the pancreas, the adrenal glands, and the gonads (ovaries and testes). Some examples of hormones are estrogens (governing female sexual development) and androgens (male hormones, including testosterone). Estrogens and progesterone are secreted by the ovaries and the adrenal glands. Testosterone is secreted by the testes.

Our knowledge of these glands is increasing. For example, today when women have a hysterectomy, the optimal choice is not to remove the ovaries. It seems that ovaries play a role that goes beyond reproduction, and unless a woman is at risk of ovarian cancer, it is better not to remove them. We also know that hormones are produced and released by other parts of the body, for example, the brain, heart, lungs, kidneys, liver, and thymus.

There is much that we have to rethink about the endocrine system and how it works. Much to the surprise of many, fat is also an important part of our endocrine system. This was only fully understood in 1994, when scientists discovered that the hormone leptin was produced by fat (also known as adipose) tissue. Leptin is a hormone that turns off the desire to eat in the brain. In addition, fat also produces protein hormones that influence energy metabolism. Fat is much more complicated than we ever imagined.

We are just learning about the different kinds of fat. There are at least two kinds of fat: (1) White fat (white adipose tissue, or WAT) stores energy, and (2) brown fat (brown adipose tissue, or BAT) burns energy to generate heat. White fat is what gives us big bellies and big rear ends. It was only a few decades ago that it was believed that only infants had brown fat, but now we know that adults also have brown fat. It is still a mystery as to what causes the development of one kind of fat instead of another.

The relationship between the immune system and the endocrine system is important in understanding diabetes. (See "Immune system and diabetes" on page 96.)

CAUSES AND PREVENTION

Beginning at the moment of conception and throughout your life, the endocrine system regulates all the processes that make your body function. The hormones your body produces are the messengers that make sure your brain, nervous system, and male or female reproductive organs develop in healthy ways; that your body can properly absorb and use food; that you grow in a systematic manner; that your blood sugar levels are healthy; and much more.

Q ***Do I have a problem?***

Maybe. If you do, you may want to include an endocrinologist (a physician who specializes in the endocrine system) among your health care providers.

Genetic defects and diabetes

Que pasa?

There are two major types of genetic defects that can cause diabetes: (1) genetic defects of the beta cells and (2) genetic defects in insulin action. Other genetic conditions associated with diabetes include Down syndrome, Klinefelter's syndrome, Huntington's chorea, porphyria, and Prader-Willi syndrome.

Causes and prevention

When diabetes is due to a defect, mutation, or change in just one gene, it is called monogenetic diabetes. The two types of monogenetic diabetes are identified by the age at which a diagnosis is first made. Neonatal diabetes mellitus (NDM) is found in infants under 6 months of age; maturity-onset diabetes of the young (MODY) is seen in adolescents or young adults. Although MODY is considered a monogenetic diabetes, it is caused by more than one gene mutation. In both conditions, the level of blood glucose is high because there is an inability to produce insulin.

Other types of genetic defects alter the ability of cells to use insulin, which results in high blood glucose levels.

Do I have a problem?

Your health care provider will give you information about the diagnosis of NDM or MODY. Among other conditions in which individuals show a defect in insulin use are acanthosis nigricans, which is identified by patches of very dark skin, and polycystic ovary syndrome (PCOS). Women with PCOS may have irregular periods, increased body hair, acne, and weight gain.

Q *What do I do now?*
Your health care provider will give you a treatment plan to follow.

Gestational diabetes

Q *Que pasa?*
A woman who did not have diabetes before develops diabetes during her pregnancy. This is more likely to happen to Hispanic women than to non-Hispanics.

CAUSES AND PREVENTION

The cause of gestational diabetes remains unknown. The concerns are for the health of the baby and for the future health of the woman. If your diabetes is untreated or uncontrolled, your baby could be born very large, have low blood glucose right after birth, or have problems breathing.

You could also develop high blood pressure during your pregnancy. Additionally, having a large baby increases the chances that you will have to have a cesarean section. About 40 to 60 percent of the women who develop gestational diabetes will develop diabetes (usually type 2) within the next 10 years. Although most women are tested between weeks 24 and 28 of their pregnancy, Latinas are usually tested earlier than that.

Q *Do I have a problem?*

According to NIDDK, at your first prenatal visit you should talk to your health care provider about being checked for gestational diabetes if any of the following statements are true:

- I have a parent, brother, or sister with diabetes.
- I am African American, American Indian, Asian American, Hispanic/Latino, or Pacific Islander.
- I am 25 years old or older.
- I am overweight.
- I have had gestational diabetes in the past.
- I have given birth to at least one baby weighing more than 9 pounds (4kg).
- I have been told that I have pre-diabetes, impaired glucose tolerance, or impaired fasting glucose.

Q *What do I do now?*

In most cases, gestational diabetes is treated by helping you be more consistent and thoughtful about the food you eat and your level of physical activity. Your health care team will give you suggestions for healthy eating and for physical activities, taking into account your lifestyle, overall health, and abilities. The 10-Point Program is a good guide to use. When it comes to managing your diabetes, remember that your goal is to control your blood glucose levels. To do this you have to eat on a regular basis; be careful about how and what you eat by watching your carbohydrate, starch, and sugar consumption; and not eat in excess.

Some women may need to take insulin to control the level of glucose in their blood. Insulin is safe because it does not get into your baby's bloodstream.

Hypoglycemia

ALSO KNOWN AS

low blood glucose or low blood sugar

Q *Que pasa?*

This is when your blood sugar levels drop below 70. When it is very severe, you can pass out.

Causes and prevention

Your blood sugar level may drop for many reasons, including taking too many medicines to lower your blood glucose level; not eating at the right time or skipping a meal; increasing physical activity without properly adjusting medicines, food, or drinks; and drinking alcohol. The impact of alcohol can be delayed 1 or 2 days, especially if you drank alcohol and had not eaten for a while. Hypoglycemia is more common in people with type 1 diabetes.

Q *Do I have a problem?*

The signs of low blood sugar vary by individual. You may feel shaky, confused, irritable, hungry, or tired. Some people get a headache while others sweat a lot. You need to know the symptoms and the signs that your body gives you when your blood sugar level is too low.

Q *What do I do now?*

If you do not have diabetes, you should see your health care provider and provide details on how you felt.

People with diabetes should be monitoring themselves on an ongoing basis. Check your blood glucose, and if it is less than 70, you need to boost the sugar in your body quickly by having one of the following:

- 1/2 cup (4 ounces [100ml]) of any fruit juice or soft drink (no diet or low calorie drinks)
- 1 cup (8 ounces [200ml]) milk
- 5 or 6 pieces of hard candy
- 1 tablespoon (15ml) of sugar or honey
- 3 or 4 glucose tablets
- 1 serving of glucose gel—the amount equal to 15 grams of carbohydrates

After you have eaten your choice from the above list, wait 15 minutes then check your blood glucose level again. If your blood glucose level is still too low, then have another serving, wait 15 minutes, and test your blood glucose level again. Keep doing this until you reach a blood glucose level of 70 or higher.

Immune system and diabetes

Q *Que pasa?*

Type 1 diabetes is an autoimmune disease. An autoimmune disease is a disease in which your immune system malfunctions and attacks your own cells. Most of the time we do not know why this occurs, but the end result is an attack by the immune system against innocent cells, like the insulin-producing cells of the pancreas. To understand this, you need to know how the immune system works.

The immune system is your personal bodyguard against microbes, bacteria, injury, viruses, and any foreign material that tries to invade your body. At the simplest level, it protects all that is "you" from all the molecules, microbes, and materials that are "not you" but try to enter your body.

Throughout your body, the immune system has different outposts set up to protect you by either keeping out or seeking and destroying invaders. These outposts include your tonsils and adenoids; the lymph nodes and the attached lymphatic vessels in your throat, armpits, and the inner leg area; the thymus (in the middle of your chest); the spleen (on your left side just above where your elbow touches); the appendix (on your right side halfway between your elbow and your wrist); Peyer's patch (left of the belly button); and throughout all your bones in the bone marrow. We are just learning about these organs. It is only recently that there was evidence that your appendix serves as a holding area to release an army of cells when called upon by the immune system to protect you.

The immune system produces a variety of cells that destroy, penetrate, or attack other cells. When you sneeze, cough, produce mucus, or have a temperature above 98.6 degrees Fahrenheit (37°C), your immune system is doing its work. Other strategies that your immune system can use to get rid of invaders include inflammation, vomiting, diarrhea, fatigue, and cramping. In some cases, once your body has been invaded by a microbe, your immune system keeps the information about what it did to protect you. Your body retains this information to use if there is another attack in the future. In a future attack, your body will launch the same defenses that proved successful in the past. Some microbes, however, are able to adapt and change themselves and in a future attack find a different way to enter your body.

Autoimmune diseases include rheumatoid arthritis and lupus.

Causes and prevention

We are learning more and more about the immune system as we have the technology to look at cells and are learning the effects that different factors as well as genes have on cells. The relationship between the immune system and the endocrine system is being studied.

Q *Do I have a problem?*

Recently, researchers have learned that when people have excess weight, it activates the immune system and makes them susceptible to inflammatory disease. When people are underweight, the immune system is suppressed and that makes them susceptible to infection and disease.

Insulin resistance

Que pasa?

Your body produces insulin but cannot use it properly. Insulin is made by the pancreas and is essential for the body to be able to use glucose for energy. Glucose is the form of sugar that is the body's main source of energy.

You eat to provide your body with the nutrition that is necessary to function. The job of your digestive system is to transform the food you eat into the nutrients that your body needs and into a form that your cells can use. Some food you eat is broken down into glucose that then travels in your bloodstream. This is known as blood glucose or blood sugar.

As you eat, the level of your blood sugar goes up. At this point your pancreas releases more insulin so that cells can absorb and use the glucose. When you have insulin resistance, your muscle, fat, and liver cells have problems absorbing the glucose and the body responds by making more and more insulin. Over time, the pancreas cannot keep up with the demand for insulin and the glucose accumulates in the bloodstream. As a result there is a high level of insulin and glucose in the bloodstream.

Causes and prevention

The exact cause of insulin resistance is not known. Various factors are known to specifically increase the likelihood of insulin resistance. Some of these we cannot change (such as genes that increase the likelihood of developing insulin resistance), but others we can manage by implementing the 10-Point Program (reducing excess weight and increasing physical activity, for example).

Q *Do I have a problem?*
The only way to know for sure is to get tested.

Metabolic syndrome

ALSO KNOWN AS
insulin resistance syndrome or syndrome X

Q *Que pasa?*
Metabolic syndrome is the name given to a group of risk factors that put you at an increased risk for heart disease, stroke, and type 2 diabetes.

CAUSES AND PREVENTION.
The cause is unknown. About 27 percent of all people in the United States have metabolic syndrome.

Q *Do I have a problem?*
Look at the risk factors below and check off the ones you have.

- ☐ You carry too much weight in your belly area. For men this means a waist larger than 40 inches (102cm), and for women larger than 35 inches (89cm).

- ☐ Your triglycerides are high. The level of triglycerides in your blood is above 150 milligrams per deciliter (mg/dL), or you are taking medicines for elevated triglyceride levels.
- ☐ Your HDL "good" cholesterol level is low. Low for men is below 40 mg/dL and for women (below 50 mg/dL). You are also at risk if you are taking medicines because you have low levels of HDL.
- ☐ Your blood pressure is high or you are taking medicine to reduce your blood pressure. A high blood pressure level is 130/85 or above.
- ☐ Your fasting blood glucose level is 100 mg/dL or above, or you are taking medicine to control your level of blood glucose.

If you checked at least 3 of the above risk factors, then it is likely you have metabolic syndrome. You should discuss your answers to the above with your health care provider.

Q *What do I do now?*

To delay the onset of diabetes, coronary heart disease, or other problems, it would be good to lose 10 percent of your body weight and start a program of physical activity. The physical activity should be of moderate intensity, and you should do it for at least 30 minutes each time. The goal would be to do it every day. You should seriously consider starting the 10-Point Program. This plan will encourage you to take your medicines and gain control over body.

Pre-diabetes

ALSO KNOWN AS
impaired fasting glucose, or IFG, impaired glucose tolerance, or IGT

Que Pasa?

Your blood glucose levels are higher than normal but not high enough for a diagnosis of diabetes. This is a very common condition. In 2007 the U.S. government estimated that 57 million people had pre-diabetes. It means you are at risk of developing type 2 diabetes and that it would be good to implement the 10-Point Program.

Causes and prevention

The cause is unknown.

Do I have a problem?

Most people have no symptoms. You will have to be tested to know if you have pre-diabetes. Everyone over 45 should be tested for diabetes. If you are under 45, you should be tested if you are overweight and have at least 1 or more of the following risk factors:

- You are physically not very active.
- A parent, brother, or sister has diabetes.
- Your blood pressure is above 140/90, or you are being treated for high blood pressure.
- Your HDL (good cholesterol) is less than 35 mg/dL.
- Your triglyceride level is above 250 mg/Dl.

- You have a history of problems with your heart or blood vessels.
- You gave birth to a baby over 9 pounds (4kg).
- You have been diagnosed with gestational diabetes, impaired fasting glucose (IFG), or impaired glucose tolerance (IGT).
- You have polycystic ovarian syndrome (PCOS).
- You have a dark velvety rash around the neck, armpits, elbows, knees, or knuckles. This rash is also called acanthosis nigricans.

You are diagnosed with pre-diabetes if your fasting plasma glucose test (FPG) is 100–125 mg/dL or your oral glucose tolerance test result is 140–199 mg/dL.

Q *What do I do now?*

If you are diagnosed with pre-diabetes, there is much that you can do to avoid getting diabetes. Following the 10-Point Program will help you realign your life to be healthier. Evidence from the Diabetes Prevention Program shows that people who lose 5 to 7 percent of their weight and increase their physical activity (walk at least 30 minutes 5 days a week) can prevent the onset of diabetes. If you have pre-diabetes, you should get your blood glucose levels checked every year.

Type 1 diabetes

ALSO KNOWN AS

insulin-dependent diabetes or juvenile diabetes

Que pasa?

Type 1 diabetes is an autoimmune disorder. In this disease, the immune system is not working well and instead of protecting the body, it attacks part of the body and destroys its own insulin-producing beta cells in the pancreas. The progressive loss of these cells means that, eventually, the pancreas is unable to produce sufficient insulin. Without insulin, cells cannot use the glucose that is in the bloodstream. This is a major problem, as glucose is the energy source for cells, and when cells cannot use glucose they malfunction and die. Additionally, since the cells cannot use the glucose, too much glucose is left in the bloodstream, making it difficult for the body to function, which leads to other problems.

CAUSES AND PREVENTION

The cause is unknown. People with type 1 diabetes account for 5–10 percent of all diagnosed cases of diabetes. There is no way to prevent type 1 diabetes.

Q *Do I have a problem?*

The symptoms usually appear over a short period and include:

- being very thirsty
- having to urinate a lot more than usual
- feeling as if you are hungry all the time
- losing weight without trying to do so
- vision that is blurry
- feeling extremely tired

If you have any of these symptoms, you should discuss it with your health care provider. Untreated type 1 diabetes is very dangerous, as a person may go into a life-threatening diabetic coma (diabetic ketoacidosis).

To determine whether or not you have type 1 diabetes, you will be given the tests described in the Diagnosis section (see page 78). You are diagnosed with diabetes if your fasting plasma glucose test (FPG) is 126 mg/dL or more or your oral glucose tolerance test is 200 mg/dL or more. To be diagnosed with type 1 diabetes, you will need an additional blood test.

Q *What do I do now?*

With all the recent medical advances, people with type 1 diabetes can now expect to live a longer life than ever before. Consistent and thoughtful action with respect to food, physical activity, medicine, and monitoring is essential. The 10-Point Program is a good guide as to what you can do to live a healthier and longer life with type 1 diabetes. Since people with type 1 diabetes cannot produce insulin, you must get insulin either by injection or by an insulin pump.

The NIDDK supported a major study called the Diabetes Control and Complications Trial (DCCT). This study found that intensive glucose control in people with type 1 diabetes resulted in preventing or delaying damage to the small blood vessels in the eyes, kidneys, and nerves.

Type 1.5 diabetes

ALSO KNOWN AS

latent autoimmune diabetes in adults, or LADA, or double diabetes

---

Q *Que pasa?*

This is when a person has symptoms of both type 1 and type 2 diabetes. According to NIDDK, up to 10 percent of people with type 2 diabetes have LADA. There are some researchers who believe that people with LADA really have a kind of type 1 diabetes that develops slowly.

Causes and prevention

The cause is unknown. The symptoms usually appear after age 30. At first, people diagnosed with LADA are still producing insulin and do not require insulin injections. After a few years of controlling their diabetes, they need to take insulin because their immune system has attacked and destroyed the beta cells in the pancreas that make insulin.

Q *Do I have a problem?*
Your health care provider needs to tell you whether you have diabetes and, if so, which type. People with LADA also have antibodies against the insulin-producing beta cells in the pancreas.

Type 2 diabetes

ALSO KNOWN AS
non-insulin-dependent diabetes and adult-onset diabetes

> I was watched for at least 5 or 10 years because diabetes runs in my family. For many years, I was told I had pre-diabetes. Then in 2006 the endocrinologist diagnosed me as having diabetes, type 2. I take one medicine twice daily, and I give myself injections twice daily. I exercise, watch what I eat, and check my blood sugar three times a day. I try to stay away from white starches—white potatoes, white bread, regular pasta—and I eat mostly whole wheat. I limit my fruits as well. —Laurie

---

Q *Que pasa?*
Most people (90–95 percent) who have diabetes have type 2 diabetes. In type 2 the body does not respond properly to the insulin that is produced by the pancreas.

Causes and prevention

The cause is unknown. Based on some very good research, there are steps that we can take to prevent type 2 diabetes.

These are all part of the 10-Point Program. You may want to expand on the 10-Point Program by specifying as a goal that you want to:

- Lose at least 5–7 percent of your body weight (if you weigh 200 pounds [91kg], that is 10 to 14 pounds [4.5–6.4kg])
- Be physically active for 30 minutes a day, 5 days a week.
- Make healthier food choices.
- Limit the amount of calories and fat in your diet.

Do I have a problem?

It is hard to know unless you get screened. Some people who have diabetes do not have any symptoms. The symptoms of type 2 diabetes include feeling tired or ill, being thirsty all the time, frequent urination especially at night, weight loss, blurred vision, frequent infections, and slow-healing wounds. These may develop so gradually that they may not even be noticeable.

When you look at risk factors, there are very few that you can change. The factors you cannot change but that may predispose you to diabetes include the following:

- You have a family history of diabetes.
- You are 45 years old or older.
- You had diabetes while pregnant (gestational diabetes).
- You have high blood pressure.
- You have polycystic ovary syndrome (PCOS).
- You have acanthosis nigricans, characterized by dark, thick, velvety patches of skin around the neck and armpits.

The risk factors that you can change are being overweight or obese and not getting enough physical activity.

Q *What do I do now?*

The most important step for you to take is to follow the plan developed by your health care team. The 10-Point Program is also a good way for you and your family to live healthier lives. If you have type 2 diabetes, you can reduce the likelihood that you will have complications from uncontrolled diabetes by doing all you can to control your diabetes. Keep in mind that if you do not control your diabetes, the onset of complications may be sudden and will make it less likely that you will be able to do the things you enjoy.

Part Three

RESOURCES AND TOOLS TO HELP YOU TAKE CONTROL

If you have questions about diabetes or any other health question, please call the National Hispanic Family Health Help Line at 866-783-2645, or 866-Su-Familia. Health promotion advisors are available to answer your questions and help you find local services. You can call the help line Monday through Friday, from 9 A.M. to 6 P.M. ET.

About Me: My Numbers from My Health Care Provider

My Blood Type ____________ **Allergies** ______________________________

Date	Blood Pressure	Weight	HDL	LDL	Total Cholesterol	Triglycerides	AIC	Procedures & Results
	/							
	/							
	/							
	/							
	/							
	/							
	/							
	/							
	/							
	/							
	/							
	/							
	/							
	/							
	/							
	/							

About Me: On a Daily Basis

Target Level ________ **Special notes** ________________

Date	Breakfast	A.M. Snack	Lunch	P.M. Snack	Dinner	Late Snack	Physical Activity
/ /							
NOTES							
/ /							
NOTES							
/ /							
NOTES							
/ /							
NOTES							
/ /							
NOTES							
/ /							
NOTES							
/ /							
NOTES							
/ /							
NOTES							
/ /							
NOTES							
/ /							
NOTES							
/ /							
NOTES							
/ /							
NOTES							

Visits to My Health Care Provider and Support Team

Date ____________________ **Why I Went** ______________________________

Whom I Saw ____

____

Special Tests ____

____

Diagnosis ____

____

Referred Elsewhere ____

____

Medicines Prescribed ____

____

What Else Did the Health Care Provider Do/Say? ____________________

____

____

____

Date ____________________ **Why I Went** ______________________________

Whom I Saw ____

____

Special Tests ____

____

Diagnosis ____

____

Referred Elsewhere ____

____

Medicines Prescribed ____

____

What Else Did the Health Care Provider Do/Say? ____________________

____

____

____

My Medicines, Supplements, Teas, and Other Things I Take

Name __________ Cost __________

Purpose __________

Size/Amount __________ Color __________ Shape __________

Date Prescribed __________ By __________

How Much Do I Take? __________ When? __________

Things to Avoid __________

Side Effects/Other Comments __________

Name __________ Cost __________

Purpose __________

Size/Amount __________ Color __________ Shape __________

Date Prescribed __________ By __________

How Much Do I Take? __________ When? __________

Things to Avoid __________

Side Effects/Other Comments __________

Questions to Discuss with My Health Care Provider

Questions About a Diagnosis

1. *Can you please repeat that?*
2. *What type of diabetes do I have?*
3. *How does that change what I have to do?*
4. *Will I have to inject myself?*
5. *Is there someone who will help me plan what I eat?*
6. *Does this mean I can never have ice cream or dessert?*
7. *Will I be able to be as physically active as I have been all along?*
8. *In my work I have to be very active. Is there anything special I should do?*
9. *What else can I expect?*
10. *Do you have any information on a DVD that I can watch at home?*
11. *Do you have anything I can take home to read about this?*
12. *How often should I come back to see you?*
13. *How should I monitor my blood glucose level?*
14. *How often should I monitor my blood glucose level?*
15. *Whom can I call if I feel I am having a problem?*
16. *Will this have an impact on my ability to be sexually intimate?*

Questions About a Diagnostic Test

1. *Can you please repeat the name of the test?*
2. *What will the test show?*
3. *Where will I have the test?*
4. *Are there any risks involved?*
5. *What special preparations should I make before the test?*
6. *How long will it take?*
7. *What will happen after the test?*
8. *Is there anything else I should know?*
9. *Who will give me the results?*
10. *How long will it take to get the results?*
11. *How often do I have to have this test?*

Questions About Ongoing Management of Diabetes

1. *How am I doing?*
2. *How often should I go for an eye exam?*
3. *Do I have to a see a podiatrist?*
4. *Can I still get a pedicure?*
5. *What do I have to do if I am traveling?*
6. *Will I be able to reduce my medicines?*
7. *How will I know if my blood glucose level is too high?*
8. *How will I know if my blood glucose level is too low?*

Questions About My Medicines

1. *Do I have to take these medicines?*
2. *I am also taking:* ______________________________
   (list the medicines ______________________________
   you are taking) ______________________________
   ____
   ____
   ____
   ____
   ____
   ____
   ____
3. *Should I still take these medicines?*
4. *Are there any reported interactions between the medicines I'm currently taking and the one(s) you're prescribing?*
5. *Have there been problems with this type of medicine?*
6. *How long will I have to take this medicine?*
7. *How do I take this medicine? With food? On an empty stomach? With lots of water?*
8. *In addition to the medicine, what else do you recommend?*
9. *Are there any natural alternatives that I can take?*
10. *Are there any natural alternatives I should avoid?*

Resources with Diabetes Information

American Diabetes Association

www.diabetes.org

This not-for-profit is the premier organization offering information about diabetes for consumers and health care providers.

Centers for Disease Control and Prevention

http://www.cdc.gov/health/diabetes.htm

This government agency, which is part of the U.S. Department of Health and Human Services (DHHS), provides information on how to prevent diabetes.

Centers for Medicaid and Medicare

www.medicare.gov

This government agency, which is part of U.S. Department of Health and Human Services (DHHS), is responsible for the Medicaid program, Medicare, and a special program for people with end-stage renal disease.

National Alliance for Hispanic Health

hispanichealth.org

This not-for-profit provides information in English and Spanish for consumers and health care providers on a wide variety of health topics.

National Diabetes Education Program

ndep.nih.gov

This is a collaborative effort of the National Institutes of Health, the Centers for Disease Control and Prevention, and more than 200 public and private organizations.

National Institute of Diabetes and Digestive and Kidney Diseases

www.niddk.nih.gov

This government agency is part of the National Institutes of Health, which is part of the U.S. Department of Health and Human Services (DHHS). NIDDK provides information on the latest research on diabetes and some consumer materials.

Acknowledgments

There are many people who make the *Buena Salud*™ series possible. The entire team at Newmarket Press, especially Esther Margolis, Heidi Sachner, Keith Hollaman, and Harry Burton, have provided incredible encouragement. The board, staff, and members of the National Alliance for Hispanic Health and the Health Foundation for the Americas also nurtured the creation of the series. For this edition, Thomas Sacks, M.D., a gifted internist, provided a thorough and extensive review, and Carolina Reyes, M.D., an obstetrician and gynecologist, shared her insights.

The personal support that I need to write came from my life sisters and brothers as well as exceptional friends and include Kevin Adams, Carolyn Curiel, Msgr. Duffy, Adolph P. Falcón, Polly Gault, Paula Gomez, Ileana Herrell, Thomas Pheasant, Sheila Raviv, Carolina Reyes, Esther Sciammarella, Cynthia A. Telles, and Elizabeth Valdez. My memories and experiences with my extraordinary mother, Lucy Delgado, my cousin Deborah Helvarg, and my friend Henrietta Villaescusa are also part of this book.

Most of all I want to thank my husband, Mark, and daughter, Elizabeth, for the inspiration and affection they provide on a daily basis. Their love frames my life and gives me the emotional sustenance for everything I do.

INDEX

About the Author

JANE L. DELGADO, Ph.D., M.S., author of *The Latina Guide to Health: Consejos and Caring Answers*, is President and Chief Executive Officer of the National Alliance for Hispanic Health (the Alliance), the nation's largest organization of health and human service providers to Hispanics. She was recognized by the *Ladies' Home Journal* as one of the "Ladies We Love" in 2010 and by *WebMD* as one of its four Health Heroes of 2008 for her dedication and resilience in advocacy. Among many other awards and honors, in 2007 *People En Español* named her to the 100 Influentials in the Hemisphere.

A practicing clinical psychologist, Dr. Delgado joined the Alliance in 1985 after serving in the Immediate Office of the Secretary of the U.S. Department of Health and Human Services (DHHS), where she became a key force in the development of the landmark "Report of the Secretary's Task Force on Black and Minority Health."

At the Alliance, Dr. Delgado oversees the national staff as well as field operations throughout the United States, Puerto Rico, and the District of Columbia. She is also a trustee of the Kresge Foundation, Lovelace Respiratory Research Institute, U.S. Soccer Foundation, Northern Virginia Health Foundation, and Health Foundation for the Americas, and serves on the national advisory councils for the Paul G. Rogers Society for Global Health Research and on the National Board of Mrs. Rosalyn Carter's Task Force on Mental Health.

Dr. Delgado received her M.A. in Psychology from New York University in 1975. In 1981 she was awarded a Ph.D. in clinical psychology from SUNY Stony Brook and an M.S. in Urban and Policy Sciences from the W. Averell Harriman School of Urban and Policy Sciences. She lives in Washington, D.C., with her husband, Mark, and daughter, Elizabeth.

Founded in 1973, the **National Alliance for Hispanic Health** is the foremost science-based source of information and trusted advocate for the health of Hispanics. The Alliance represents local community agencies serving more than 15 million persons each year and national organizations serving over 100 million persons, making a daily difference in the lives of Hispanic communities and families.

The Health Foundation for the Americas (HFA) supports the work and mission of the National Alliance for Hispanic Health, and seeks individuals, companies, agencies, foundations, and sponsors to help support its programs to improve the quality of health care for all, which includes providing timely and trusted bilingual health information. Every year HFA supports programs to improve health for all by helping secure clean air to breathe, clean water to drink, safe places to play, and healthy food to eat. HFA and the Alliance help those without health care gain access to free and low-cost services where they live and improve the quality of health care. The programs put new health technology to work in communities, provide millions of dollars in science and health career scholarships, and conduct the research and advocacy that is transforming health.

Dr. Delgado's book *The Latina Guide to Health: Consejos and Caring Answers* is published simultaneously in English- and Spanish-language editions by Newmarket Press. The author is donating all royalties from the Spanish edition to the Health Foundation for the Americas.

You can be a part of this extraordinary mission of health and well-being. To learn more about the Alliance or the HFA, visit www.hispanichealth.org or www.healthyamericas.org.

Newmarket Titles by Jane L. Delgado

Written specifically for the growing U.S. Latino population by Jane L. Delgado, Ph.D., M.S., the president and CEO of the National Alliance for Hispanic Health, *The Buena Salud™ Guides* present the best in health advice, available in both English and Spanish-language editions.

The Buena Salud™ Guide to Diabetes and Your Life
Introduction by Larry Hausner, CEO, America Diabetes Association

Featuring the stories of people and families living with diabetes—a condition that has touched the lives of most Hispanic families—this concise guide explains everything readers need to know, including the important fact that diabetes is not inevitable.

The book discusses: the factors that contribute to developing diabetes and how to prevent it; the types and evolving definition of diabetes; how the endocrine and immune systems function; the impact of the environment on diabetes; treatment options, including medication and realistic changes in lifestyle and diet; and features an A-Z section with all commonly used diabetes terms.

Paperback • 128 pages • ISBN: 978-1-55704-941-4 • $9.95

Also available in Spanish:
La guía de Buena Salud™ sobre la diabetes y tu vida (978-1-55704-942-1)

The Buena Salud™ Guide for a Healthy Heart
Introduction by Jack Lewin, M.D., CEO, American College of Cardiology

Opening with a personal story from Dr. Delgado about her mother's experience with heart disease, this invaluable guide details everything readers need to know about the leading cause of death for all men and women in the U.S.

The book explains: how the heart works; how heart problems develop and what can be done to avoid them; achievable lifestyle changes to maintain heart health; and features an A-Z section with all commonly used heart terms.

Paperback • 128 pages • ISBN: 978-1-55704-943-8 • $9.95

Also available in Spanish:
La guía de Buena Salud™ para un corazón sano (978-1-55704-944-5)

ALSO BY JANE L. DELGADO, PH.D., M.S.

The Latina Guide to Health: Consejos and Caring Answers
Foreword by Antonia Novello, M.D., M.P.H., Dr.P.H., Former U.S. Surgeon General

Featuring cutting-edge medical information and advice fo all Hispanic women, Dr. Delgado offers practicial information on the health issues women face, separates myths from facts, and answers questions about what to do. She discusses arthritis, cervical cancer, depression, and other important topics in a quick-reference health section.

Paperback • 240 pages • ISBN: 978-1-55704-854-7 • $15.95

Also available in Spanish:
La guía de salud: Consejos y respuestas para la mujer latina
(ISBN: 978-1-55704-855-4)

The Buena Salud™ Guide for a Healthy Heart
______ copies at $9.95 each
La guía de Buena Salud™ para un corazón sano
______ copies at $9.95 each

The Buena Salud™ Guide to Diabetes and Your Life
______ copies at $9.95 each
La guía de Buena Salud™ sobre la diabetes y tu vida
______ copies at $9.95 each

The Latina Guide to Health: Consejos and Caring Answers
______ copies at $15.95 each
La guía de salud: Consejos y respuestas para la mujer latina
______ copies at $15.95 each

For postage and handling, add $5.00 for the first book, plus $1.50 for each additional book. Please allow 4–6 weeks for delivery. Prices and availability subject to change.

I enclose a check or money order, payable to Newmarket Press, in the amount of $__________. (New York State residents, please add applicable sales tax.)

Name ____

Address ______________________________________

City/State/Zip _________________________________